CONGRATULATIONS ON YOUR DECISION TO GET HEALTHY!

Twenty-One Healthy Ice Pop Snack Recipes

COOKBOOK VII

A guide to a *new healthy "frozen-snacks" recipe plan* that is not a "DIET", created based on personal experience to help you *finally* keep up with your weight loss management, weight management and overall health goals.

ALSO BY KYLA LATRICE, MBA

"New Me, New You! (How I Overcame Obesity)"

"The 7 Day Smoothie Detox"

"The 21 Day Slushie & Juice Fast"

"The 21 Day Salad Fast"

"Eat Well and Stay Thin (Living a Healthy You)"

"21 Days to a New Healthy You! Hearty Vegan & Vegetarian
Slow Cooker Recipes"

"Twenty-One Healthy Ice Pop Snack Recipes"

"21 Days of Everyday Healthy Snack Recipes"

"All Natural Soups & Stews"

"A Collection of My Favorite Health Recipes"

"A New You! Workout Workbook"

"21" HEALTHY ICE-POP
Snack Recipes

A 21 DAY ICE-POP SNACK RECIPE GUIDE BASED ON MY BOOK "21 DAYS TO A NEW HEALTHY YOU: DRINK YOUR WAY THIN! (SMOOTHIE FAST)"; TO HELP YOU STAY ON TRACK WITH YOUR WEIGHT MANAGEMENT AND HEALTH GOALS with the fun of "snack rewards" for a better *"LIFE"*

KYLA LATRICE, MBA

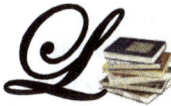

Lady Mirage Publications, Inc.

New York   Memphis   Los Angeles   London   Cape Town   Toronto
Atlanta   Singapore   Japan

Published by:
Lady Mirage Publications, Inc.
3724 Goodman Rd W, Unit 575
Horn Lake, MS 38637
www.LadyMirageAgency.com

Manufactured in the United States of America
First Edition: September 2014

Lady Mirage Publications, Inc. is an imprint and subsidiary
of Lady Mirage Global. The Lady Mirage Publications, Inc. name
and logo are trademarks of Lady Mirage Global.

Authors within the Lady Mirage Global (under Lady Mirage Agency,
Inc.), Lady Mirage Publications and Lady Mirage Literary Agency
speakers division provides a wide range of authors for speaking
engagements. To find out more information, go to
www.LadyMirageAgency.com
Cover photo provided by www.FreeDigitalPhotos.net
The publisher is not responsible for websites (or their content) that
are not owned by the publisher.

Library of Congress Cataloging-in-Publication Data:
eISBN: 978-1-31-120132-4; Print ISBN: 978-0-9975371-6-1
Tennin, Kyla Latrice.
Twenty-One Healthy Ice Pop Snack Recipes
Pages cm; copyrighted materials.
1.   Health-Nutrition-Diet-Fitness. 2. Cooking. 3. Fitness.
Library of Congress Catalog Card Number: 2016907239

Print Book Edition, License Note

Also Note

In this book, Ms. Latrice begins by explaining a *fast* that she has created, tested and tried, which contributed to her weight loss, weight management and healthy eating lifestyle journey. She has also written this book due to there being so many books, health, weight-loss and "diet" programs currently on the global market. The programs and books she has seen and reviewed are too long, too thick, have too much information and many times, are difficult for people to read. This book was written to ***simplify and shorten*** how to lose weight and maintain your health, for life. It is based on personal experience and is still done today. It's an effective solution.

TWENTY-ONE HEALHTY ICE POP
SNACK RECIPES

Table of Contents

DEDICATION

This cookbook is dedicated to men and women around the world that have dealt with or are beginning to deal with food addiction, obesity and/or declining health.

I also dedicate this book to those whom have been "Mirage's" in life; overlooked, betrayed, not good enough, slandered, mistreated, misunderstood, misrepresented and even treated unfairly because of their weight or how they looked on the *outside* to others, when in fact, on the *inside* there's greater.

This new cookbook is also dedicated to men and women around the world that want to
shift from being ordinary to extraordinary and accomplishing what others said you would never be able to do again or never be able to do at all.

Here's to the New You!

ACKNOWLEDGMENTS

I want to *say thank you* to anyone whom has ever betrayed,
rejected, mistreated, teased, and misused
or looked down upon me. You helped me become GREATER
and launched me into my destiny.

Whenever someone throws bricks at you, use them to *"build"*.
Build something greater; even your mansion.

And whenever you face opposition, "know" that it is actually
an opportunity; a set-back for a set-up to secure the victory,
rejection for rewards, pain for gain, lack for prosperity to
leave a legacy, misery for miracles and put downs for
promotion.

IT'S YOUR TIME...*to bounce back!*

Let's Get Healthy!

AUTHOR'S NOTE

AFFIDAVIT

All content written herein is of opinion, from personal experience and of suggestion. Individual Ice Pop Recipes and new eating plan results may vary from person to person and no results are guaranteed.

You must put forth effort and do the work necessary to take charge of changing your life and *losing weight*. I did and so can you.

You can also utilize this cookbook if you have already met your weight loss goals and just want to stay healthy with recipes that will keep your metabolism in check and body running smoothly.

Be sure to wash all fruits, vegetables, foods, etc. thoroughly before beginning any new eating or meal plan.

ALL RIGHTS RESERVED

"ON-THE-GO"

This cookbook *(and all of my cookbooks,*
books, workbook and manuals) can be read and applied in
airports, on trains, at work on your lunch break,
in grocery stores while shopping for and planning your
weekly meals, at bookstore cafes,
at restaurants *(for quick decision making; to remember your*
health and/or weight loss goals) and even in shopping malls.

In addition, *this book can be brought to*
fast food restaurants (to pull up and look through to remember
your goals before ordering), at the park (before a jog or
potluck), during your hotel stays,
on vacations and at airport food counters when ordering your
meals and drinks *(so you remember your goals and what to*
eat and drink).

This cookbook has been made available
on mobile devices via Adobe Digital Editions and DRM
(Digital Rights Management).

WORLD STATISTICS

Obesity and Childhood Obesity
Centers for Disease Control and Prevention
http://www.cdc.gov/obesity/data/adult.html
http://www.cdc.gov/nchs/fastats/obesity-overweight.htm

Harvard School of Public Health
http://www.hsph.harvard.edu/obesity-prevention-source/obesity-trends/

World Health Organization
http://www.who.int/topics/obesity/en/

Stroke Awareness and Prevention
http://www.cdc.gov/stroke/facts.htm

Diabetes Awareness and Prevention
Centers for Disease Control and Prevention
http://www.cdc.gov/diabetes/data/statistics/2014statisticsreport.html

American Diabetes Association
http://www.diabetes.org/diabetes-basics/statistics/

"FASTING"

WHAT IS FASTING?

➢ Fasting is abstaining from PLEASURABLE foods for a certain amount of time to FOCUS on things that are more important than pleasurable foods to get to the root of what is causing your poor health, obesity, relationships and quality of life.

➢ It is not a hunger strike.

➢ You're able to see into your life better and rid it of the bad when you pull away from portion after portion at the dinner table, lunch buffet after buffet with friends and co-workers, nightly binge eating and drinking (whether alcohol, sodas, sugary drinks and the like) and dessert or movie nights on the sofa with a large pizza box and donuts.

➢ Fasting helps you pinpoint where you overdo things (overindulge), gets you back on track and teaches you how to eat, "in moderation" (balance), for your health and for a better life.

➢ Your body may not like eating healthy for the first few days (especially if you have never fasted before), but it will adjust.

REASONS FOR FASTING:

➢ It produces a physical discipline (especially for how, when, where and *what* you eat).

➢ It rids the body of toxins (just like exercise does when you sweat); cleansing your body and digestive tracts, improving your health and weight.

Note: If you are on medication, consult your physician before any *fast*.

BENEFITS OF FASTING:

➢ It strengthens *you* and your body.

➢ Fasting brings joy, happiness and *energy* to your life; and fruits, vegetables, oils, etc. are quite inexpensive. Make a list and shop for your ingredients before you begin.

➢ You become very aware of *what* and *how much* you eat. You also begin to pay more attention to when and where you always eat/drink and what leads you to OVEREATING.

➢ Fasting brings humility, revelation and an overall healthy lifestyle (mind, emotions, intellect, etc.).

TYPICAL TYPES OF FASTS:

Sometimes people fast the following from their lives:

➢ Television (even the internet, social media or video games) for one day, three days or even one week, television during certain hours of the day (to break a cycle of watching certain shows they may be addicted to (like food) that aren't good for them.

.....or

➢ To break a cycle of "certain foods" they may eat while watching certain television shows.

➢ Fasting to abstain from all pleasurable foods and red meats, eating only fruits, vegetables, clear soups, cereals (no white sugar), water, diluted fruit juices (100% juices only) and/or grains.

➢ Some people even fast people (bad acquaintances, friendships or relationships), leading eventually to moving away from those person's completely, for a better life and health. Your health is your life.

- Many people fast for 24 hours, three days, seven days, 14 days, 21 days or longer. My success and learning my body as well as other persons bodies (whom have fasted when I have fasted) has come from "closely monitoring" how the body reacts to each of these fasts (particularly "21 days") and I've noticed some things and have sculpted recipes to help others find that tremendous success in many areas of their lives as well.

- Fasts should always be broken slowly, especially if you have been on an "extended fast" (a fast for more than 30 days, a salad only fast, a smoothie only fast or even a clear soup only fast).

- Gradually get back into "regular food", until you can completely commit to "healthy food" (and a regular healthy lifestyle); such as having juices for a couple of days, then fruits, vegetables, grains and adding meats back into your diet last, if applicable.

- Typically, people have six meals per day (three main meals (breakfast, lunch and dinner) and three snacks). For each of my Fasts or Recipes, you determine how many meals. Don't worry, fruits and vegetables do not cause obesity, they prevent it. Yet, always watch your portion sizes, in general, and with soups, stews and anything that has meat included. Never eat meat in excess.

- You can even choose to eat one meal per day for 21 days (there are enough recipes listed in this book), a snack, have 5-8 bottles of water and be sure to get a nap in and some exercise during the week. As you advance you can mix your salad fast with a smoothie fast and detox fast by doing one of the fasts, each per week, for 21 days, etc.

THE *"SMOOTHIE FAST"* BIRTH

Kyla Latrice is a native of Marks, MS and enjoys food and traveling. Being from a small town and a country gal, she set her goals high. Graduating from a private institution with a Bachelor of Arts Degree (BA) *(women's studies and health background; pre-medicine)* and a Master's Degree (MBA) in Business Administration with **Executive Education at Harvard and Stanford** along with several certifications and nearly 50-80 self-study coursework in legal, intellectual property and self-help, she has become one of the leading entrepreneurs of her time.

Currently Ms. Latrice is finishing up her Doctoral Honorary Degree *(Doctor of Management in Organizational Leadership)* and continues to serve on Board of Directors throughout the world for various causes; still relating to her life's purpose and corporations work. Ms. Latrice travels extensively for speaking engagements in the areas of health, wellness, obesity, poverty, domestic violence, branding, image, leadership, mentoring, business, entrepreneurship and the like.

To date, Ms. Latrice has mentored with over 20 plus organizations *(from elementary to senior citizen)*, helping others overcome issues she has faced.

With her first *corporate* job opportunity being at a "Health Food Restaurant" *(when she was age 15 or 16)* to work as a deli attendant at the deli bar, hostess *(when others were out for the day)* and bakery attendant as well as a chef in the *salad bar*.

Her main role was to attend to the deli, to prepare healthy pasta salads, healthy sandwiches, healthy shakes, healthy sundaes and *healthy smoothies*. However, Ms. Latrice was blessed with the opportunity to be called upon whenever management needed her help in the other areas as well, **to continue learning**. This gave Ms. Latrice very valuable experience and a "look" into health and business ownership, a bit deeper, which still remains with her today.

THE *"SMOOTHIE FAST"* BIRTH

KYLA LATRICE
BEFORE
21 DAY SMOOTHIE FASTS

Ms. Latrice's *(on the left in the photo)* Corporations are inclusive of health restaurants, retail stores, property and land as well as product development organizations along with nonprofit foundations to care for the displaced, homeless.

Further, Ms. Latrice's love for food turned into obesity when her life took a turn in the early 2000's during domestic violence, sinful relationships, bad friendships, emotional binge eating and more; then again in the 2000's with another domestic violence relationship, obesity slander from family members, mental and spiritual abuse, abortion, home foreclosure, vehicle repossession and much *more*, which all have an effect on health, but she made sure her Corporations still stood; to help others.

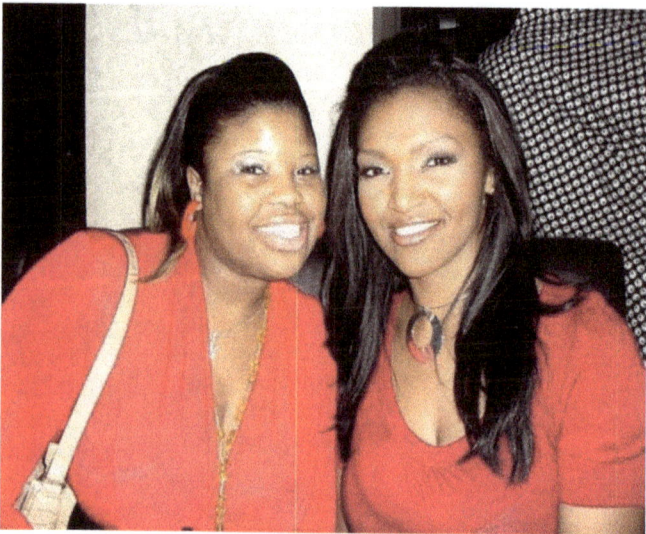

THE *"SMOOTHIE FAST"* BIRTH

KYLA LATRICE
"IN THE MIDDLE"
AFTER GAINING WEIGHT BACK FOR A SECOND TIME
21 DAY SMOOTHIE FASTS

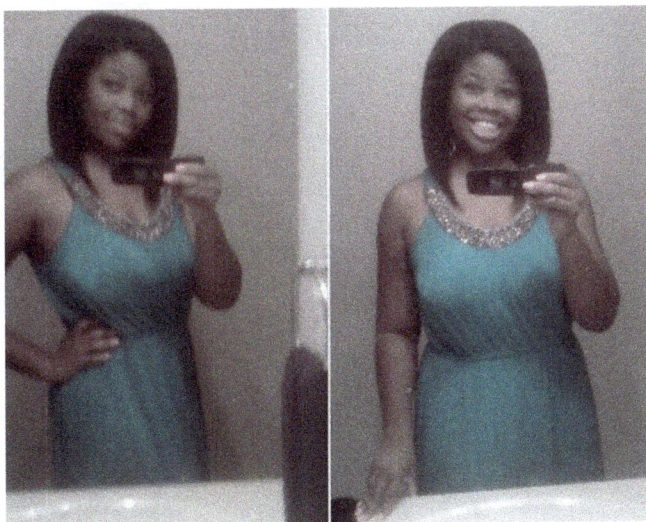

THE *"SMOOTHIE FAST"* BIRTH

KYLA LATRICE
AFTER
21 DAY SMOOTHIE FASTS

THE FINALE

Many factors can contribute to obesity, such as abuse *(mental, spiritual, physical, sexual)*, poor eating habits, environment, bad friendships, sin and more. Personally, I, myself, was never taught how to eat, I did not know what to eat *(that was truly healthy for me)* and I did not know how to deal with life's problems.

Nevertheless, how can someone teach you what they don't know? My first encounter with obesity was when I was a model and went from a size 0 to a size 20/22, **weighing close to 300 pounds** *(then I lost nearly 115 pounds after prayer and seeking a remedy)*.

The second encounter was when I gained some of the first encounters weight back and went from a size 14/16 to a size 4/6 and fitting a 7/8 in jeans, losing 68 pounds. Today, I am going to share my secrets to success with you *(the birth of the "21 Day Salad Fast")* and how I made it out over the years ***and*** kept the weight off. Let's get started and healthy, for life!

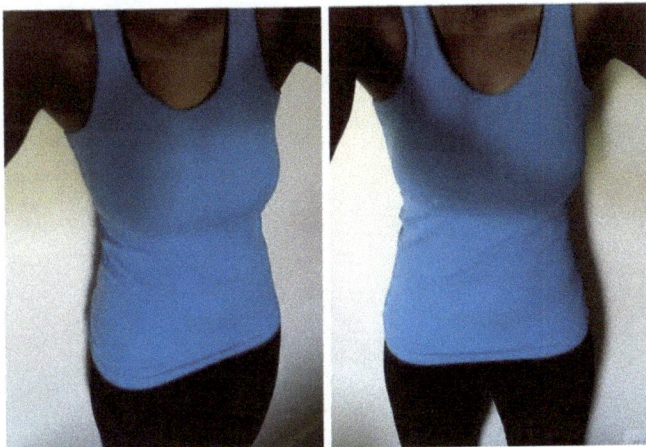

GETTING HEALTHY
LIFESTYLE CHANGE

Prepare to lose weight on the "Smoothie Fast" (this is not a "diet", this is an "eating plan" to reprogram your mind, body and metabolism about how to eat (portion control) and regarding what foods you should and should not be eating). It is designed to help you become healthier. Before starting this fast and any of my eating *plans ("The 21 Day Smoothie Fast" and "The 21 Day Salad Fast" as well as "Soups and Stews")*, allow yourself "one week" to prepare for the fast and eating plan by removing the following from your life:

➢ Negative relationships and friendships; they block you from doing well in life and succeeding, when people begin to see you doing well, they tend to not like it. Choose friendships and associations wisely. Be creative.

➢ Bad acquaintances; they will eventually want what you have and will cause betrayal to take place in your life through a "set-up" to sabotage all of your hard work. Always keep moving forward.

➢ Remove the following (slowly) from your daily meals (eating habits) because they contribute to weight gain (some quicker than others): soda, breads, pastas, candy bars and the like and eating second, third and fourth portions of your food. You only need one portion. Don't eat the rest!

➢ Replace all sodas with diet soda until you can cut soda out of your daily meal plan completely; only drink soda if absolutely necessary *(a lemon-lime beverage)* because there is nothing else to drink. For example, while traveling.

➢ Remove all "junk food" (cakes, pies, chips, all kinds of desserts and the like) from your kitchen.

➢ For breads, certain kinds make the weight gain skyrocket; be careful about pizza. Pasta should be limited just like soda, having it only if absolutely necessary, but once every 2-4 months is okay, just like donuts, to stay **balanced** and give your body a break from always eating healthy.

➢ Again, you only need one portion of food, per meal, work on this and you'll see results quicker.

➢ Increase your water intake to 5-8 bottled waters a day; bring a bottle with you everywhere you go so you'll be forced to drink it *(instead of something else)* and will program your body to like it *(whether you like it frozen, warm or cold)*.

➢ When you're out to eating with others, begin selecting items from menus that help *(not hinder)* your **new eating plan**, for example, order a "grilled chicken wrap with a side salad and small water" instead of a double cheeseburger, french fries and large soda. Never super-size, it wastes your results and time spent on improving your health.

➢ If you have not already, purchase my books: *"The 7 Day Detox"* and *"The 21 Day Salad Fast"* to begin, to continue your weight loss and new you.

➢ And again, remember, commit to single portion eating, eating smaller portions (always have more vegetables on your plate than poultry/ meat), and increase your water intake *(remember to use the restroom)*. Let's begin.

GETTING HEALTHY
SET GOALS

Feel free to purchase my "A New Healthy You Workout Workbook" *(to go with your **new eating plan** and my "fasts" cookbooks* or a composition notebook from any retailer to make your own journal to measure the following (even if you need to do so at your primary care physician's office, a free clinic or go to a free health assessment machine in a retail store location that has one):

Record a written record of each:

- ➢ Your Cholesterol Level.
- ➢ Blood Pressure and Vision Check.
- ➢ Your actual Height Weight, Height, Bust/Chest and Hips size (write down your goals of where you want to be in the next week, three months, six months and year).
- ➢ Record your weight, chest/bust, hips and waist size every Saturday morning at 7am.
- ➢ Stroll through a department store and notate clothing (or take a camera phone photo) you plan on fitting into someday and notate your current sizes and then return in three months to see how you're fairing up towards your goals.
- ➢ Pick up my *"A New Healthy You Workout Workbook"* or list in your journal, your reasons for losing weight, changing your life and changing your eating habits.

> Your BMI (Body Mass Index) and where you are versus where you're supposed to be for your height, weight, age and gender.
> Bottles of "cold water" listed in most of my books recipes sections are in reference to drinking 4-5 bottles of 16 fl oz bottles of water, which is equivalent to 8-10 glasses of water per day.
> Water is vital for living and for being healthy.
> The amount of water within the human body is typically 50-65% water and in infants, 78%.
> Water assists your body with digesting food and getting nutrients from the foods you have eaten to your blood, brain and other parts of your body, in order to function; emptying the body of waste and toxins, helps deliver oxygen to the body, helps prevent constipation and even regulates body temperature (in your cells, organs and tissues).

A (BMI) Chart is below for your convenience.

BMI	<(less than) 18.5	=	Underweight
BMI	18.5-24.9	=	Normal Weight
BMI	25-29.9	=	Overweight
BMI	>(more than) 30	=	Obese

GETTING HEALTHY
WHILE TRAVELING

If you'll be traveling by airplane, helicopter or private jet (smile):

> ➤ Research where you will be eating ahead of time (food choices, ingredients and prices).
> ➤ Bring bottled water.
> ➤ Resist vending machines and relying of fast food at your final destination.
> ➤ Bring your own snacks (trail mix, cashews, a banana, apple slices, peanuts) and
> ➤ Workout for free in your hotel room, taking the stairs instead of elevators and walking at the Mall.

If traveling by car:

> ➤ Pack your own cooler with ice for your bottled waters, fruits and raw vegetables.
> ➤ Consider bringing a bag of oranges & any other food that can be eaten warm or cold on the road.

If you'll be traveling by bus, train, or other means:

> ➤ Research where you will be eating ahead of time (food choices, ingredients and prices).
> ➤ Bring bottled water.
> ➤ Bring your own snacks (trail mix, cashews, a banana, apple slices, peanuts for the long trip) and
> ➤ Bring something to read or play, to keep your mind off of food and *fictious* hunger.
> ➤ At your destination, stand more than you sit (to keep your body moving) and since you have been sitting during traveling for your trip.

PEARS

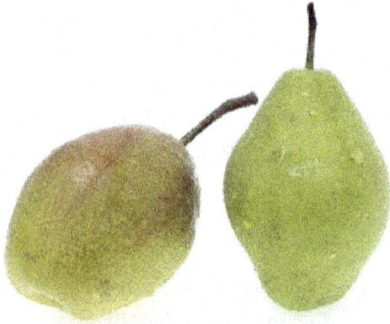

GETTING HEALTHY
YOUR NEW WORKOUT PLAN

During my both times of being obese, I never worked out at a gym nor went outside of my home to run *(weighing in at 278 pounds and trying to start my "new me" as a jogger was terrible on my knees)* to lose weight, I did it all at home, on the floor, in a compact room, near a closet. I suggest you begin a "workout regime" by doing simple workouts, such as crunches, stretching, leg lifts and a few push-ups.

Everyone cannot do cardio in the gym (paid membership prices or because of lack of transportation), running outside or bouncing around in-doors for 1-3 hours like actors and actresses on television, whom are likely being *paid monetary* compensation or by other means to film the infomercial.

Remain constant and do this 3-4 times a week, for 15-35 minutes each day. On your workout OFF days, do 100 crunches before going to bed. Consider purchasing my "Workout Workbook" to keep up with your Fitness Plan. In addition, you burn calories when you sleep, by drinking water, by exercising (which helps you live longer as well) and by **movement** (whether your arms, legs, looking out of a window, etc.).

Furthermore, water helps break down food and helps food digest. Your can also do a "mental workout" by cutting out negative people, places and things from your life.

You'll find that you have more peace in your brain and life, when you replace them with reading inspirational books, movies, community work and exercise or things you love, such as knitting, a ball game, taking a site seeing road trip (alone) every now and then or mentoring someone.

Notes

_____
_____
_____
_____
_____
_____
_____
_____
_____
_____
_____
_____
_____
_____
_____
_____
_____
_____
_____
_____
_____
_____
_____
_____
_____
_____
_____
_____

THE SIX MONTH RULE
GIVE IT *"TIME"*

THE SIX-MONTH RULE

On a 21-Day Salad Fast, weight [pounds] have been known to drop quickly for many people. However, the goal here is to also keep the weight off. Stay focused and be committed to at least six-months of "health work".

Remember to journal your progress.

There's something about when you write things down, they get *ACCOMPLISHED!* Also give yourself a total of six-months to work on your "New You" simply because you may lose inches first and not weight, until your weight catches up with your inches (this is what took place with me; loosing 10-12 pounds per month).

Inches first then one day the weight just fell off. And for others, sometimes weight first, then inches.

GO BACK TO THE DEPARTMENT STORE

Revisit those same department stores that you went to on the first week of your new lifestyle change, try on new clothing sizes to see where you are with your goals.

I suggest that you "mentally shop" for a new suit, a dinner dress, clothing for you next vacation (Hawaii maybe), your first pair of skinny jeans or baseball gear to wear to a game; all after you have reached your goals; to *CELEBRATE!*

Ice Pop Tray and Wooden Sticks Examples & where to purchase

AMAZON.COM
http://www.amazon.com/dp/B00LZM3WWA/ref=twister_B00 6MPYBV6

PASTRYCHEF.COM
http://www.pastrychef.com/ICE-CREAM-POP-MAKER_p_1857.html

Wooden Sticks (can come in many colors, typically brown)

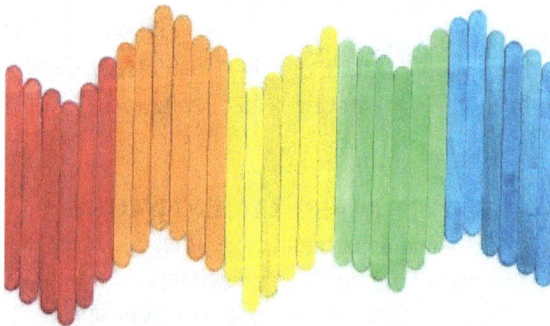

Photo Credit: aopsan
Freedigitalphotos.net

"ICE POP"
RECIPES

BLUEBERRIES

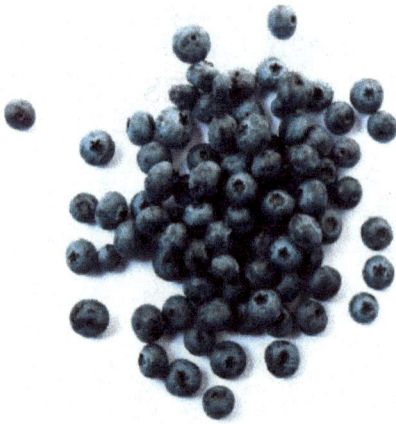

DAY 1
(SWEET BLUEBERRY DELIGHT)

Add 1 cup of frozen blueberries into a blender
Add 1 cup of frozen raspberries
Add 1 cup of ice
Add 2-3 cups of chilled 100% orange juice (no pulp)
Add a tsp of sweet honey into the blender
Blend until smooth
Pour into a glass or bullet to go blender cup or blender mug
Prepare "Ice-Pop" Tray immediately

Health Note:
Blueberries are infused with great sources of Vitamins C and E, riboflavin, niacin and folate. Blueberries also have proanthocyanidins (to help fight aging) and phytonutrients ellagic acid (anticancer protection) in them along with catechins to help burn abdominal fat to double weight loss.

Ice-Pop Snack Creation:
- ➢ Pour the smoothie base into an ice-pop tray *(that was previously set in a freezer)*
- ➢ After filling the entire tray, place the ice-pops into a freezer to freeze for about 20 minutes
- ➢ Place wooden sticks into (store bought in a bag; many dollar stores sell them as well) ice-pop trays to stand tall
- ➢ Place tray back into the freezer and freeze until hard, then enjoy.

RASPBERRIES

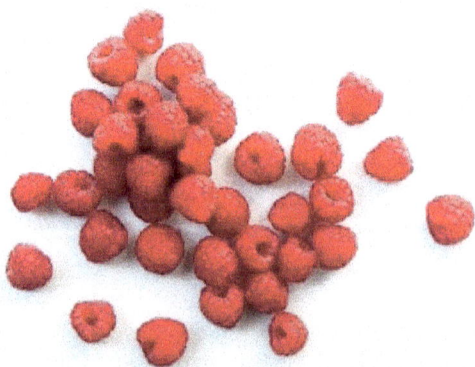

DAY 2
(RASPBERRY LOVER)

Add 1 cup of frozen raspberries into a blender
Add 1 cup of frozen strawberries
Add 1 cup of ice
Add 2-3 cups of chilled 100% apple juice
Add a tsp of sweet honey into the blender
Blend until smooth
Pour into a glass or bullet to go blender cup or blender mug
Prepare "Ice-Pop" Tray immediately

Health Note:

     Raspberries are known for having a good source of fiber, Vitamin C, manganese, Vitamin B2, folate, niacin, copper and potassium.

     They are also low in sugar (fructose) and have antioxidant to help fight illness and disease.

Ice-Pop Snack Creation:
- ➢ Pour the smoothie base into an ice-pop tray *(that was previously set in a freezer)*
- ➢ After filling the entire tray, place the ice-pops into a freezer to freeze for about 20 minutes
- ➢ Place wooden sticks into (store bought in a bag; many dollar stores sell them as well) ice-pop trays to stand tall
- ➢ Place tray back into the freezer and freeze until hard, then enjoy.

MANGOES

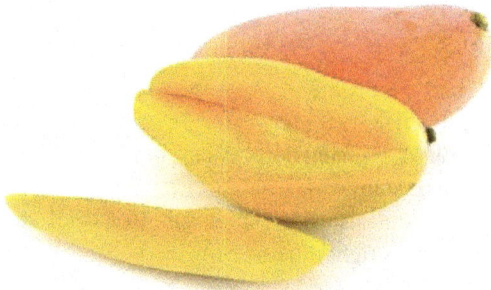

DAY 3
(MANGO MELLY JELLY)

Add 1 cup of frozen diced mangoes into a blender
Add 1 cup of frozen diced peaches
Add 1 cup of ice
Add 2-3 cups of chilled 100% orange juice (no pulp)
Add a tsp of sweet honey into the blender
Blend until smooth
Pour into a glass or bullet to go blender cup or blender mug
Prepare "Ice-Pop" Tray immediately

Health Note:
Mangoes are rich in Vitamins A (antioxidant and vision repairer) and C (antioxidant and immune booster) as well as Vitamins B6, copper, potassium, beta-carotene, magnesium and even healthy probiotic fiber.

Mangoes also help clear skin (acne and clogged pores), fight cancer, lowers cholesterol, help digestion, aids in weight loss, aids in memory and is high in iron for women.

Ice-Pop Snack Creation:
➢ Pour the smoothie base into an ice-pop tray *(that was previously set in a freezer)*
➢ After filling the entire tray, place the ice-pops into a freezer to freeze for about 20 minutes
➢ Place wooden sticks into (store bought in a bag; many dollar stores sell them as well) ice-pop trays to stand tall
➢ Place tray back into the freezer and freeze until hard, then enjoy.

LIMES

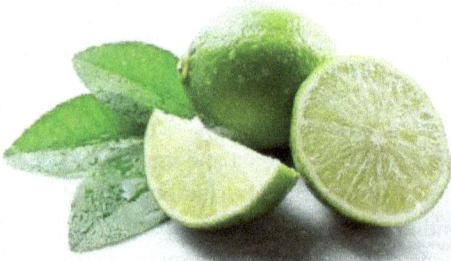

DAY 4
(LIME AND KIWI DELIGHT)

Add 1 cup of frozen kiwi into a blender
Add 1 diced lime
Add 1 cup of ice
Add 2-3 cups of chilled 100% apple juice
Add a tsp of sweet honey into the blender
Blend until smooth
Pour into a glass or bullet to go blender cup or blender mug
Prepare "Ice-Pop" Tray immediately

Health Note:
      Kiwi fruit is a small powerhouse that helps manage blood pressure because of its high level of potassium and helps with digestion.
      Kiwi is high in fiber and low glycemic index for weight loss, rich in immunity booster Vitamin C and carries Vitamin E for clearer skin; also fighting heart disease and cleaning toxins from the body.

Ice-Pop Snack Creation:
- ➢ Pour the smoothie base into an ice-pop tray *(that was previously set in a freezer)*
- ➢ After filling the entire tray, place the ice-pops into a freezer to freeze for about 20 minutes
- ➢ Place wooden sticks into (store bought in a bag; many dollar stores sell them as well) ice-pop trays to stand tall
- ➢ Place tray back into the freezer and freeze until hard, then enjoy.

STRAWBERRIES

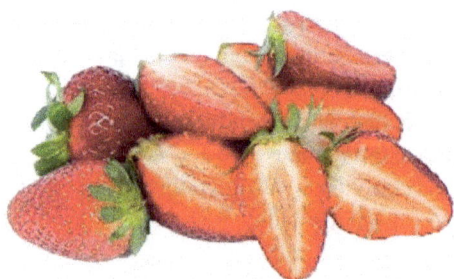

DAY 5
(STRAWBERRY MANGO, RASPBERRY BLUES)

Add 1 cup of frozen strawberries into a blender
Add 1 cup of frozen diced mangoes
Add 1 cup of frozen raspberries
Add 1 cup of ice
Add 2-3 cups of chilled 100% apple juice
Add a tsp of sweet honey into the blender
Blend until smooth
Pour into a glass or bullet to go blender cup or blender mug
Prepare "Ice-Pop" Tray immediately

Health Note:

Strawberries improve blood sugar regulation and are high in fiber and help BURN stored fat. They are packed with antioxidants (like Vitamin C) to help fight wrinkles and ease Inflammation. They also contain Vitamin K, potassium and magnesium.

Nitrate is also included in these sweet honey bees for weight loss.

Ice-Pop Snack Creation:

➢ Pour the smoothie base into an ice-pop tray *(that was previously set in a freezer)*

➢ After filling the entire tray, place the ice-pops into a freezer to freeze for about 20 minutes

➢ Place wooden sticks into (store bought in a bag; many dollar stores sell them as well) ice-pop trays to stand tall

➢ Place tray back into the freezer and freeze until hard, then enjoy.

CANTALOUPE

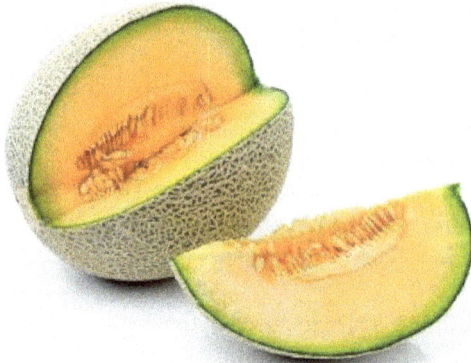

DAY 6
(CANTALOUPE CRANBERRY SWEETHEART)

Add 1 cup of frozen diced cantaloupe into a blender
Add 1 cup of frozen cranberries
Add 1 cup of ice
Add 2-3 cups of chilled 100% orange juice (no pulp)
Add a tsp of sweet honey into the blender
Blend until smooth
Pour into a glass or bullet to go blender cup or blender mug
Prepare "Ice-Pop" Tray immediately

Health Note:
Cranberries are high in fiber and Vitamin C, helping the kidneys and to prevent urinary tract infections (UTIs). They also have no fat and no sodium making them a favorite for those with bladder problems.
Cranberries also help fight tooth decay and boost the immune system. Cranberry Juice flushes out your system and speeds up weight loss with antioxidants.

Ice-Pop Snack Creation:
➢ Pour the smoothie base into an ice-pop tray *(that was previously set in a freezer)*
➢ After filling the entire tray, place the ice-pops into a freezer to freeze for about 20 minutes
➢ Place wooden sticks into (store bought in a bag; many dollar stores sell them as well) ice-pop trays to stand tall
➢ Place tray back into the freezer and freeze until hard, then enjoy.

PINEAPPLE

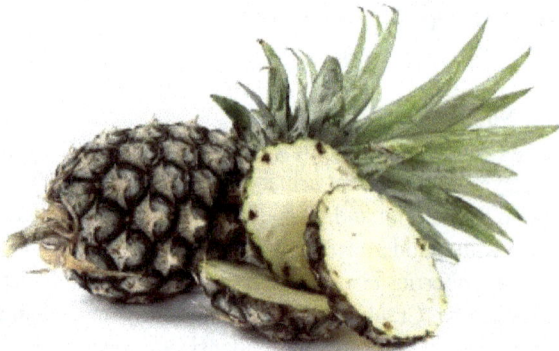

DAY 7
(PINEAPPLE BANANA TRUTH)

Add 1 cup of frozen diced pineapple into a blender
Add ½ cup of (non-frozen) sliced banana
Add 1 cup of ice
Add 2-3 cups of chilled 100% orange juice (no pulp)
Add a tsp of sweet honey into the blender
Blend until smooth
Pour into a glass or bullet to go blender cup or blender mug
Prepare "Ice-Pop" Tray immediately

Health Note:
Bananas strengthen your blood to prevent anemia and are high in iron and calcium (to prevent calcium loss during urination; drinking lots of water will cause urination) as well as potassium (aiding in weight loss and preventing stroke).

Bananas strengthen your bones, fight depression and muscle cramps and are a great source of Vitamin B-6.

Ice-Pop Snack Creation:
- ➢ Pour the smoothie base into an ice-pop tray *(that was previously set in a freezer)*
- ➢ After filling the entire tray, place the ice-pops into a freezer to freeze for about 20 minutes
- ➢ Place wooden sticks into (store bought in a bag; many dollar stores sell them as well) ice-pop trays to stand tall
- ➢ Place tray back into the freezer and freeze until hard, then enjoy.

WATERMELON

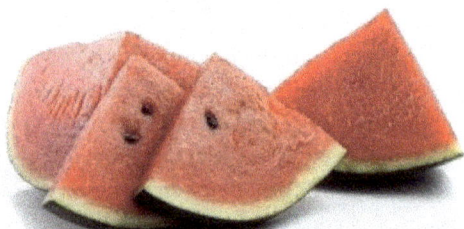

DAY 8
(WATERMELON STRAWBERRY PASSION)

Add 1 cup of frozen diced (seedless) watermelon into a blender
Add 1 cup of frozen strawberries
Add 1 cup of ice
Add 2-3 cups of chilled 100% orange juice (no pulp)
Add a tsp of sweet honey into the blender
Blend until smooth
Pour into a glass or bullet to go blender cup or blender mug
Prepare "Ice-Pop" Tray immediately

Health Note:

Watermelon is a plant that is originally from Southern Africa. Its fruit is a special berry that has a ripe source of Vitamins C, A, D, B-12, beta carotene, thiamin, B-6. Iron, Calcium, potassium and magnesium are also included.

Watermelon is low in calories and aids in wound healing, stress relief and quenching cravings to assist with weight loss.

Ice-Pop Snack Creation:
- ➢ Pour the smoothie base into an ice-pop tray *(that was previously set in a freezer)*
- ➢ After filling the entire tray, place the ice-pops into a freezer to freeze for about 20 minutes
- ➢ Place wooden sticks into (store bought in a bag; many dollar stores sell them as well) ice-pop trays to stand tall
- ➢ Place tray back into the freezer and freeze until hard, then enjoy.

GRAPEFRUIT

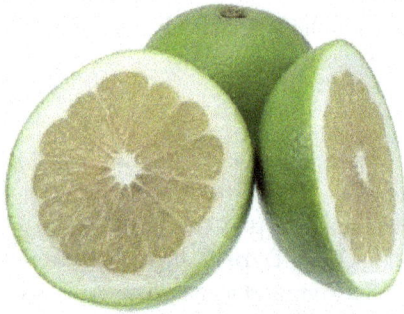

DAY 9
(GRAPEFRUIT WATERMELON SWEETNER)

Add 1 cup of frozen diced grapefruit into a blender
Add 1 cup of frozen diced watermelon
Add 1 cup of ice
Add 2-3 cups of chilled 100% apple juice
Add a tsp of sweet honey into the blender
Blend until smooth
Pour into a glass or bullet to go blender cup or blender mug
Prepare "Ice-Pop" Tray immediately

Health Note:

Grapefruit is naturally full of water and fiber and helps you stay full longer. It also battles aging and fights the common cold and flu. Vitamins included in this beauty are Vitamins C, A, E as well as K.

Grapefruit also helps lower cholesterol levels. The fruit also aids in fighting insomnia, fatigue, fevers and digestive disorders.

Ice-Pop Snack Creation:
➢ Pour the smoothie base into an ice-pop tray *(that was previously set in a freezer)*
➢ After filling the entire tray, place the ice-pops into a freezer to freeze for about 20 minutes
➢ Place wooden sticks into (store bought in a bag; many dollar stores sell them as well) ice-pop trays to stand tall
➢ Place tray back into the freezer and freeze until hard, then enjoy.

RASPBERRIES

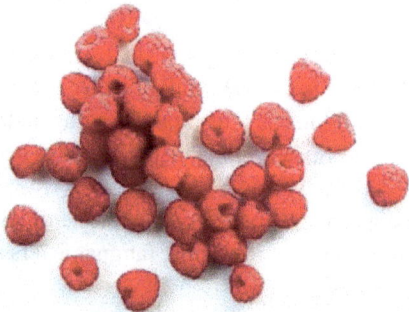

DAY 10
(RASPBERRY PINEAPPLE BLUEBERRY FIX)

Add 1 cup of frozen raspberries into a blender
Add 1 cup of frozen diced pineapple
Add 1 cup of frozen blueberries
Add 1 cup of ice
Add 2-3 cups of chilled 100% grapefruit juice
Add a tsp of sweet honey into the blender
Blend Until smooth
Pour into a glass or bullet to go blender cup or blender mug
Prepare "Ice-Pop" Tray immediately

Health Note:
        Pineapples can be found in the Caribbean, Southern Brazil, Paraguay, Hawaii, Philippines and even Costa Rica. Being rich in Vitamin C, this fruit helps boost the immune system and aids in reducing arthritis pain.
        Pineapple helps promote strong bones, healthy gums, fights bronchitis, high blood pressure and Macular Degeneration (vision loss).

Ice-Pop Snack Creation:
  ➤ Pour the smoothie base into an ice-pop tray *(that was previously set in a freezer)*
  ➤ After filling the entire tray, place the ice-pops into a freezer to freeze for about 20 minutes
  ➤ Place wooden sticks into (store bought in a bag; many dollar stores sell them as well) ice-pop trays to stand tall
  ➤ Place tray back into the freezer and freeze until hard, then enjoy.

BLACKBERRIES

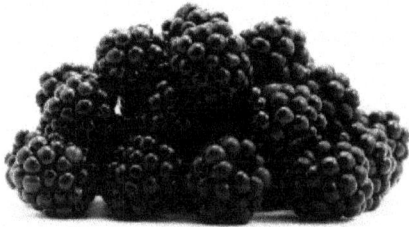

DAY 11
(CHILLED BLACKBERRY STRAWBERRY FIX)

Add 1 cup of frozen blackberries into a blender
Add 1 cup of frozen diced strawberries
Add 1 cup of ice
Add 2-3 cups of chilled 100% apple juice
Add a tsp of sweet honey into the blender
Add a squeeze of a lemon's fresh juice
Blend until smooth
Pour into a glass or bullet to go blender cup or blender mug
Prepare "Ice-Pop" Tray immediately

Health Note:
 Blackberries are special. They help your skin continue to look younger, keeps your brain alert, reduces inflammation of your gums and relaxes your muscles.
 These berries also help prevent colon cancer (with their Vitamins E and C) and oral cavities.

Ice-Pop Snack Creation:
  ➤ Pour the smoothie base into an ice-pop tray *(that was previously set in a freezer)*
  ➤ After filling the entire tray, place the ice-pops into a freezer to freeze for about 20 minutes
  ➤ Place wooden sticks into (store bought in a bag; many dollar stores sell them as well) ice-pop trays to stand tall
  ➤ Place tray back into the freezer and freeze until hard, then enjoy.

ORANGES

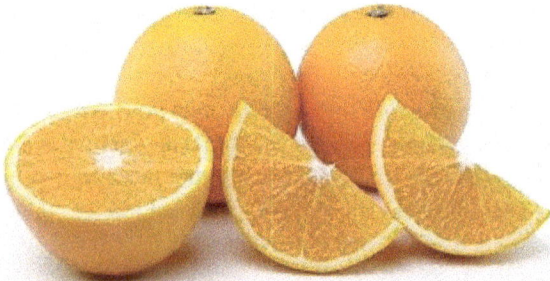

DAY 12
(ORANGE STRAWBERRY DUE BERRY)

Add 1 cup of non-frozen, peeled oranges into a blender
Add 1 cup of frozen diced strawberries
Add 1 cup of ice
Add 2-3 cups of chilled 100% apple juice
Add a tsp of sweet honey into the blender
Add a squeeze of a lemon's fresh juice
Blend until smooth
Pour into a glass or bullet to go blender cup or blender mug
Prepare "Ice-Pop" Tray immediately

Health Note:

Oranges are rich in potassium and Vitamin C.
Oranges help regulate blood pressure, aid in relieving
constipation, infections, risk of liver cancer, kidney stones and
lowers cholesterol.

This fruit is also rich in citrus limonoids, which have
proved to fight a number of varieties of cancers inclusive of:
skin, lung, breast, stomach and colon.

Ice-Pop Snack Creation:

➢ Pour the smoothie base into an ice-pop tray *(that was previously set in a freezer)*
➢ After filling the entire tray, place the ice-pops into a freezer to freeze for about 20 minutes
➢ Place wooden sticks into (store bought in a bag; many dollar stores sell them as well) ice-pop trays to stand tall
➢ Place tray back into the freezer and freeze until hard, then enjoy.

GRANOLA

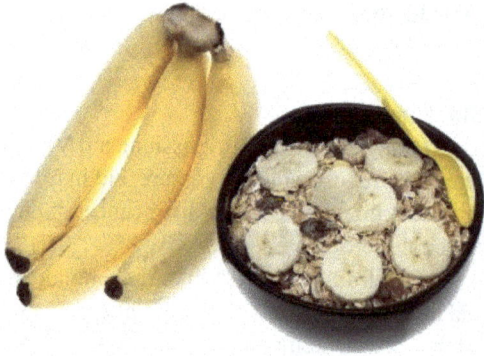

DAY 13
(STRAWBERRY BANANA GRANOLA GLORY)

Add 1 cup of frozen strawberries into a blender
Add ½ cup of (non-frozen) sliced banana
Add ½ cup of diced granola
Add a tsp of white protein powder
Add 1 cup of ice
Add 2-3 cups of chilled 100% orange juice (no pulp)
Add a tsp of sweet honey into the blender
Blend until smooth
Pour into a glass or bullet to go blender cup or blender mug
Prepare "Ice-Pop" Tray immediately

Health Note:
     A small portion of Granola goes a long way. This oat has ingredients of dried fruit, nuts and coconut.
     The dried fruit in granola provides additional fiber in your smoothies, promoting digestive health. Oats are a great source of Vitamin E, selenium, magnesium, copper, zinc, magnesium and iron.

Ice-Pop Snack Creation:
➢ Pour the smoothie base into an ice-pop tray *(that was previously set in a freezer)*
➢ After filling the entire tray, place the ice-pops into a freezer to freeze for about 20 minutes
➢ Place wooden sticks into (store bought in a bag; many dollar stores sell them as well) ice-pop trays to stand tall
➢ Place tray back into the freezer and freeze until hard, then enjoy.

GINGER

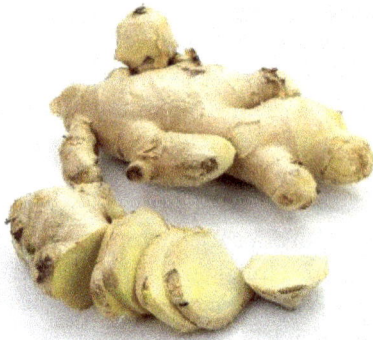

DAY 14
(GINSENG STRAWBERRY WONDER)

Add 1 cup of frozen strawberries into a blender
Add ½ cup of (non-frozen) sliced banana
Add a tsp of ginseng or ginger *(a small portion goes a long way)*
Add 1 cup of ice
Add 2-3 cups of chilled 100% orange juice (no pulp)
Add a tsp of sweet honey into the blender
Blend until smooth
Pour into a glass or bullet to go blender cup or blender mug
Prepare "Ice-Pop" Tray immediately

Health Note:
Ginseng includes extracts that have berries that aid in weight control (working as a natural appetite suppressant), fighting obesity. It also aids in lessening stomach pain linked to menstrual cramps.

Ginseng also helps reduce stress, boosts the immune system, fights colds, gives you energy, improves your mood and treats hepatitis C and high blood pressure.

Ice-Pop Snack Creation:
➢ Pour the smoothie base into an ice-pop tray *(that was previously set in a freezer)*
➢ After filling the entire tray, place the ice-pops into a freezer to freeze for about 20 minutes
➢ Place wooden sticks into (store bought in a bag; many dollar stores sell them as well) ice-pop trays to stand tall
➢ Place tray back into the freezer and freeze until hard, then enjoy.

TANGERINES

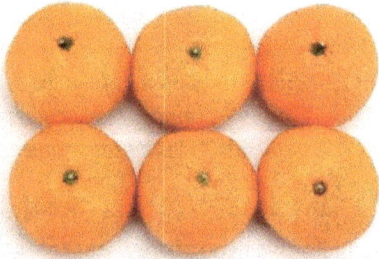

DAY 15
(THE TANGERINE TANGO)

Add 1 cup of frozen diced tangerines into a blender
Add 1 cup of frozen strawberries
Add a tsp of white protein powder
Add 1 cup of ice
Add 2-3 cups of chilled 100% apple juice
Add a tsp of sweet honey into the blender
Blend until smooth
Pour into a glass or bullet to go blender cup or blender mug
Prepare "Ice-Pop" Tray immediately

Health Note:

Tangerines are Mandarin Oranges that aid in fighting obesity, keeping your heart healthy and fighting against the development of diabetes. Tangerines are rich in Vitamin A, potassium and folate (a B-Vitamin).

These beauties help heal minor cuts and wounds, fight skin diseases & arthritis, promotes Hair Growth & Delays Hair Greying and improves digestion.

Ice-Pop Snack Creation:
- ➢ Pour the smoothie base into an ice-pop tray *(that was previously set in a freezer)*
- ➢ After filling the entire tray, place the ice-pops into a freezer to freeze for about 20 minutes
- ➢ Place wooden sticks into (store bought in a bag; many dollar stores sell them as well) ice-pop trays to stand tall
- ➢ Place tray back into the freezer and freeze until hard, then enjoy.

PEACHES

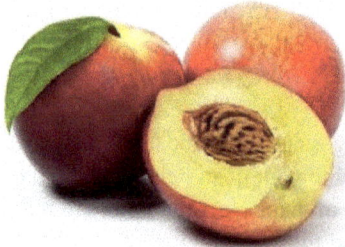

DAY 16
(SWEET PEACH PASSION)

Add 1 cup of frozen peaches into a blender
Add 1 cup of ice
Add 2-3 cups of chilled 100% orange juice (no pulp)
Add a tsp of sweet honey into the blender
Blend until smooth
Pour into a glass or bullet to go blender cup or blender mug
Prepare "Ice-Pop" Tray immediately

Health Note:
     Peaches are a great fruit that also help fight obesity
by keeping you fuller longer; *controlling* your weight.
     They contribute to keeping your eyes healthy,
prevent cancer and hair loss, aid in cleansing your kidneys,
bladder and toxins from the body. Also, they are rich in
Vitamins A and C as well as a mineral that aids in cell damage
protection.

Ice-Pop Snack Creation:
> ➢ Pour the smoothie base into an ice-pop tray *(that was previously set in a freezer)*
> ➢ After filling the entire tray, place the ice-pops into a freezer to freeze for about 20 minutes
> ➢ Place wooden sticks into (store bought in a bag; many dollar stores sell them as well) ice-pop trays to stand tall
> ➢ Place tray back into the freezer and freeze until hard, then enjoy.

HONEYDEW MELON

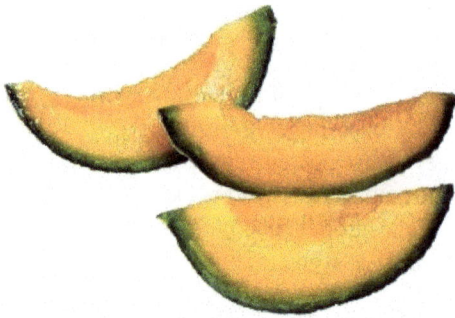

DAY 17
(TROPICAL HONEYDEW MELON PASSION)

Add 1 cup of frozen diced honeydew melon into a blender
Add 1 cup of frozen diced apricot
Add 2 tsp of a shot of wheat grass
Add 1 cup of ice
Add 2-3 cups of chilled 100% grapefruit juice
Add a tsp of sweet honey into the blender
Blend until smooth
Pour into a glass or bullet to go blender cup or blender mug
Prepare "Ice-Pop" Tray immediately

Health Note:
        Honeydew Melons are a white fruit *(can also be orange in color)* with the size and look of a Cantaloupe. Vitamins in honeydew melons are A, C, D, K, E, B-6, B-12, Niacin, Thiamin, Riboflavin and even D-3. Honeydew melons originated in Southern France and Algeria.
        Honeydew aids in boosting levels of collagen for younger looking skin, aids in vision and controlling blood pressure.

Ice-Pop Snack Creation:
  ➤ Pour the smoothie base into an ice-pop tray *(that was previously set in a freezer)*
  ➤ After filling the entire tray, place the ice-pops into a freezer to freeze for about 20 minutes
  ➤ Place wooden sticks into (store bought in a bag; many dollar stores sell them as well) ice-pop trays to stand tall
  ➤ Place tray back into the freezer and freeze until hard, then enjoy.

PEARS

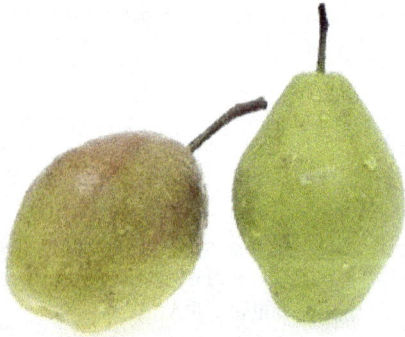

DAY 18
(PINEAPPLE PASSION)

Add 1 cup of frozen diced pineapple into a blender
Add ½ of a (non-frozen) diced pear
Add 1 cup of ice
Add 2-3 cups of chilled 100% white grape juice
Add a tsp of sweet honey into the blender
Blend until smooth
Pour into a glass or bullet to go blender cup or blender mug
Prepare "Ice-Pop" Tray immediately

Health Note:

Pears come in many shapes sizes and colors. The most common color is green. Also, pears help reduce risk of cancer and prevent high blood pressure, helps with constipation, osteoporosis, shortness of breath and gives energy.

They are also packed with fiber and promote a well body, fighting sickness.

Ice-Pop Snack Creation:
- ➤ Pour the smoothie base into an ice-pop tray *(that was previously set in a freezer)*
- ➤ After filling the entire tray, place the ice-pops into a freezer to freeze for about 20 minutes
- ➤ Place wooden sticks into (store bought in a bag; many dollar stores sell them as well) ice-pop trays to stand tall
- ➤ Place tray back into the freezer and freeze until hard, then enjoy.

KIWI

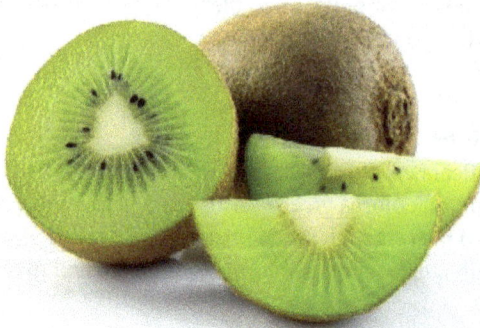

DAY 19
(WATERMELON KIWI TWIST)

Add 1 cup of frozen diced watermelon into a blender
Add 1 cup of (non-frozen) diced kiwi
Add 1 cup of ice
Add 2-3 cups of chilled 100% acai berry juice (with pulp)
Add a tsp of sweet honey into the blender
Blend until smooth
Pour into a glass or bullet to go blender cup or blender mug
Prepare "Ice-Pop" Tray immediately

Health Note:

The secret ingredient in this smoothie is "Acai Berry" juice. Acai berries are known for aiding in lowering cholesterol levels, increasing overall heart health.

The acai **oil** in the berry helps with generating healthy skin and the **pulp** in the berry aids in weight loss and fighting obesity. Acai berries also boost energy and mental function.

Ice-Pop Snack Creation:

➤ Pour the smoothie base into an ice-pop tray *(that was previously set in a freezer)*
➤ After filling the entire tray, place the ice-pops into a freezer to freeze for about 20 minutes
➤ Place wooden sticks into (store bought in a bag; many dollar stores sell them as well) ice-pop trays to stand tall
➤ Place tray back into the freezer and freeze until hard, then enjoy.

PLUMS

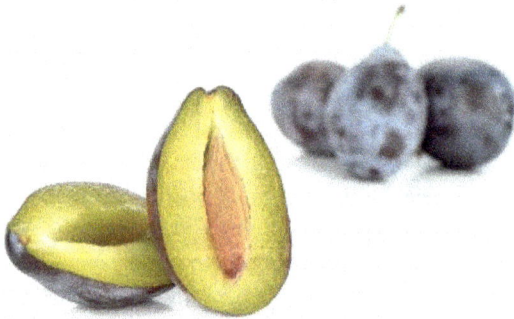

DAY 20
(STRAWBERRY JELLY BELLY)

Add 1 cup of frozen strawberries into a blender
Add ½ of a (non-frozen) diced plum
Add 1 cup of ice
Add 2-3 cups of chilled 100% white grape juice
Add a tsp of sweet honey into the blender
Blend until smooth
Pour into a glass or bullet to go blender cup or blender mug
Prepare "Ice-Pop" Tray immediately

Health Note:
        Plums (similar to prunes) are rich in B-6. They help
reduce high blood pressure and reduce stroke risk, due to their
potassium content. In addition, plums contain potassium,
fluoride and iron as well as Vitamins A, C and K.
        They help remove toxins from the body, fight the
development of diabetes and aid in maintaining regular
bowels.

Ice-Pop Snack Creation:
  ➤ Pour the smoothie base into an ice-pop tray *(that was
    previously set in a freezer)*
  ➤ After filling the entire tray, place the ice-pops into a
    freezer to freeze for about 20 minutes
  ➤ Place wooden sticks into (store bought in a bag;
    many dollar stores sell them as well) ice-pop trays to
    stand tall
  ➤ Place tray back into the freezer and freeze until hard,
    then enjoy.

KIWI

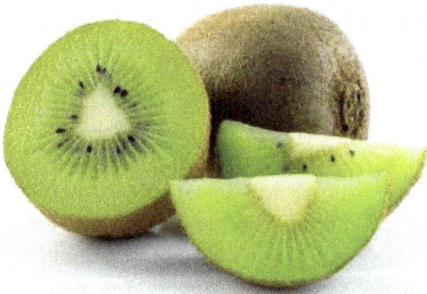

DAY 21
(PINEAPPLE KIWI POWERHOUSE)

Add 1 cup of frozen diced pineapple into a blender
Add 1 cup of (non-frozen) diced kiwi
Add 2 tsp of a shot of wheat grass *(the organic powder or the juiced grass if you have a juicer)*
Add 1 cup of ice
Add 1 cup of chilled 100% apple juice
Add 1 cup of chilled 100% orange juice (no pulp)
Add a tsp of sweet honey into the blender
Blend until smooth
Pour into a glass or bullet to go blender cup or blender mug
Prepare "Ice-Pop" Tray immediately

Health Note:
      Wheatgrass juice contains up to 70% chlorophyll, which helps build blood (increased hemoglobin production).
      Wheatgrass also helps prevent the graying of hair, helps with joint pain, bladder issues, removes toxins from the liver, fights cancer, arthritis, acne, scars, dandruff and detoxes the body.

Ice-Pop Snack Creation:
- ➢ Pour the smoothie base into an ice-pop tray *(that was previously set in a freezer)*
- ➢ After filling the entire tray, place the ice-pops into a freezer to freeze for about 20 minutes
- ➢ Place wooden sticks into (store bought in a bag; many dollar stores sell them as well) ice-pop trays to stand tall
- ➢ Place tray back into the freezer and freeze until hard, then enjoy

CONGRATULATIONS ON YOUR NEW YOU!

*Keep up the great work by continuing
on with my two newest books, "The 21 Day Smoothie Fast"
and the "21 Day Salad Fast"*

INDEX OF RECIPES